Keto Soup Cookbook 2021

Ketogenic Fat Burning Soups For Your Keto Lifestyle

Kaylee LOPEZ

TABLE OF CONTENTS

Mozzarella Tomato & Basil Soup

Servings: 6

Preparation time: 15 minutes

Cooking Time: 30 minutes

INGREDIENTS

- 4 cups vegetable broth
- 1 cup canned tomatoes, diced
- 1 cup mozzarella cheese, shredded
- 1 cup heavy cream
- 1 yellow onion, chopped
- 2 garlic cloves, peeled

DIRECTIONS

1. Basil, freshly chopped for serving
2. Take a stockpot and add all the Ingredients except basil, cheese and heavy cream into it.
3. Place stockpot over medium heat.
4. Let it bring to a boil.
5. Reduce heat to simmer for 30 minutes.
6. Warm the heavy cream during the soup is cooking.
7. Blend until smooth by using an immersion blender.
8. Stir in the mozzarella cheese.
9. Garnish with fresh basil.
10. Serve and enjoy!

NUTRITION: Calories: 122; Total Fat: 9g; Protein: 6g; Carbs: 5g

Cream of Asparagus & Parmesan Soup

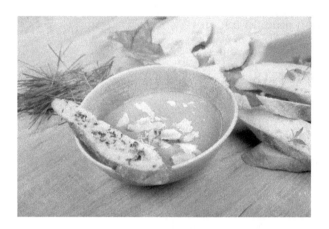

Servings: 4

Preparation time: 10 minutes Cooking

Time: 15 minutes

INGREDIENTS

- 2 cups chicken broth
- 1 cup Parmesan cheese, shredded
- 1 cup heavy cream
- 1 teaspoon thyme, dried
- 1 cup asparagus, finely chopped
- 1 yellow onion, chopped
- 3 garlic cloves, peeled
- Salt & Black pepper, to taste

DIRECTIONS

1. Take a stockpot and add all the Ingredients except Parmesan cheese and heavy cream into it.
2. Let it bring to a boil.
3. Simmer for 10 minutes.
4. Warm the heavy cream and then add to the soup along with the parmesan cheese.
5. Stir until the cheese has softened.
6. Serve and enjoy!

NUTRITION: Calories: 228; Total Fat: 17g; Protein: 12g; Carbs: 7g

Greek Lemon and Chicken Soup

Servings: 4

Preparation time: 15 minutes Cooking Time:

15 minutes **INGREDIENTS**

- The original Greek chicken soup with an added flavor of lemon.
- 2 cups chicken, cooked and chopped
- 2 cans of chicken broth, fat-free
- 2 medium carrots, chopped
- ¼ teaspoon ground black pepper
- 2 tablespoons parsley, snipped
- ¼ cup lemon juice
- 1 can cream of chicken soup, fat-free and low sodium
- ½ cup onion, chopped
- 1 clove garlic, minced

DIRECTIONS

1. Take a pot and add all the Ingredients except parsley into it.
2. Season with salt and pepper.
3. Bring the mix to a boil over medium-high heat.
4. Reduce the heat and simmer for 15 minutes.
5. Garnish with parsley.

6. Serve hot and enjoy!

NUTRITION: Calories: 582;   Total Fat: 33g;
Protein: 31g; Carbs: 33g

. Leek & Cauliflower Soup

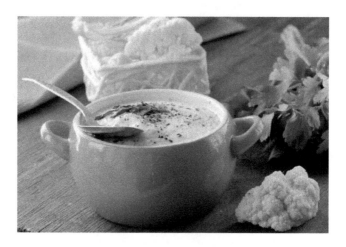

Servings: 6

Preparation time: 10 minutes Cooking Time:
40 minutes

INGREDIENTS

- A leek and cauliflower soup don't have to be bland, and this is the definitive proof of it!
- 3 cups cauliflower, riced
- 1 bay leaf
- 1 teaspoon herbs de Provence
- 2 garlic cloves, peeled and diced
- ½ cup full-fat coconut milk
- 2 and ½ cups vegetable stock
- 1 tablespoon coconut oil

- ¼ teaspoon cracked pepper
- 1 leek, chopped

DIRECTIONS

1. Take a pot, heat oil into it.
2. Sauté the leeks in it for 5 minutes.
3. Add in the garlic and then stir cook for another minute.
4. Add all the remaining Ingredients and mix them well.
5. Cook for 30 minutes.
6. Stir occasionally.
7. Blend the soup until smooth by using an immersion blender.
8. Serve hot and enjoy!

NUTRITION: Calories: 90; Total Fat: 6.4g; Protein: 1.6g; Carbs: 4.5g

. Garlic Mushroom & Beef Soup

Servings: 6

Preparation time: 10 minutes Cooking

Time: 40 minutes **INGREDIENTS**

- 1 pound beef chuck, cubed
- 6 cups chicken broth
- 1 and ½ cups cremini mushrooms
- ½ cup heavy cream
- ½ cup whipped cream cheese
- 2 teaspoons ginger, grated
- 1 yellow onion, chopped
- 2 garlic cloves, peeled
- Salt and pepper, to taste
- 1 tablespoon coconut oil, for cooking

DIRECTIONS

1. Take a skillet, add the coconut oil and brown the beef.
2. Take a stockpot and add the beef first and then all the Ingredients except heavy cream into it.
3. Mix them well.
4. Place stockpot over medium heat.
5. Let it bring to simmer and whisk again to mix cream cheese with the soup.
6. Cook for 30 minutes.
7. Then warm the heavy cream and mix with the soup.

8. Serve and enjoy!

NUTRITION: Calories: 315; Total Fat: 19g; Protein: 30g; Carbs: 5g

Broccoli Cheese Soup

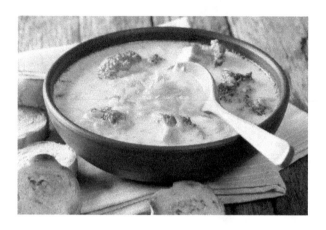

Servings: 6

Preparation time: 5 minutes

Cooking Time: 6 hours and 15 minutes

INGREDIENTS

- 4 cups broccoli, cut into florets
- 3 cups cheddar cheese
- 1 cup heavy cream
- 3 and ½ cups of chicken broth
- Salt, garlic, onion powder, and pepper, to taste

DIRECTIONS

1. Add all Nutritional Info   per Serving: to a crockpot.
2. Close the lid.

3. Cook for 6 hours on low.

4. Now open the lid and add cheese.

5. Cook for 15 minutes on high with closed lid.

6. Remove the bay leaves.

7. Make a smooth puree by using a blender.

8. Serve hot and enjoy!

NUTRITION: Calories: 291; Total Fat: 25g; Protein: 15g; Carbs: 5g

. Friendly Cucumber Soup

Servings: 4

Preparation time: 15 minutes Cooking

Time: nil **INGREDIENTS**

- 2 tablespoons garlic, minced
- 4 cups English cucumber, peeled and diced
- ½ cup Greek yogurt, plain
- ½ cup onions, diced
- 1 tablespoon lemon juice
- 1 and ½ cups vegetable broth
- ¼ cup parsley, diced
- ¼ teaspoon red pepper flakes
- ½ teaspoon salt

DIRECTIONS

1. Add all the listed Ingredients except cucumber to blender.
2. Blend until smooth.
3. Top with extra cucumbers.
4. Serve and enjoy!

NUTRITION: Calories: 169; Total Fat: 12g; Protein: 3g; Carbs: 6g

Lamb and Herb Bone Broth

Preparation Time: 10 minutes

Cooking time 8 hours

Servings: 6

INGREDIENTS

- 1 lb lamb bones
- 1 tbsp olive oil
- 1 onion, diced
- 3 celery sticks, roughly chopped
- 3 garlic cloves
- 3 sprigs rosemary
- 5 sprigs thyme
- 3 gallons of water
- Salt to taste

DIRECTIONS

1. Preheat oven to 3900F.
2. Place the lamb bones in a roasting pan and roast for 40 minutes or until browned.
3. Add oil in a saucepan and sauté onions, celery, garlic cloves, rosemary, and thyme for 5 minutes.

4. Transfer the sautéed onion mixture to the slow cooker then add the lamb bones.

5. Add 1 gallon of water and cook for 8-24 hours on Low, uncovered, making sure you add water when the level drops.

6. Use a fine-mesh strainer to strain the broth through.

7. Serve and enjoy when hot.

NUTRITION: Calories 52, Total Fat 4g, Saturated Fat 2g, Total Carbs 1g, Net Carbs 1g, Protein 3g, Sugar: 0.3g, Fiber: 0g, Sodium: 56mg, Potassium: 470mg

Chili Coney Dog Sauce

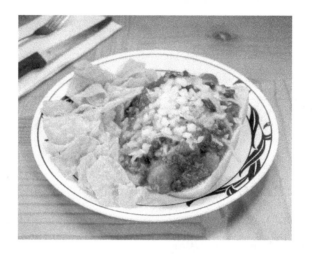

Preparation Time: 20 minutes

Cooking time 4 hours

Servings: 8

INGREDIENTS

- 1 lb. ground beef, extra lean

- 15 oz tomato sauce

- ½ cup water

- 1 ½ tbsp Worcestershire sauce

- ¼ cup onion, minced

- 1 tbsp mustard, ground

- ½ tbsp garlic powder

- ½ tbsp black pepper, freshly ground

- ½ tbsp chili powder
- ⅛ tbsp cayenne pepper

DIRECTIONS

1. Cook beef in skillet until it's no longer pink. Break the beef into crumbles then drain it.
2. Add the cooked beef to the slow cooker with the rest of the Ingredients.
3. Cover the slow cooker and cook on low for 4 hours.
4. Serve the sauce as a hot dog topping. Enjoy.

NUTRITION: Calories 118, Total Fat 6g, Saturated Fat 2g, Total Carbs 4g, Net Carbs 1g, Protein 12g, Sugar: 3g, Fiber: 1g, Sodium: 83mg, Potassium: 210mg

1. Cucumbers Pork Broth

Preparation Time: 10 minutes

Cooking time 6 hours Servings: 4

INGREDIENTS

- 1 pork butt roast, bone-in
- 1 onion, peeled and quartered
- 12 baby cucumbers
- 2 celery stalks, halved
- 4 ½ cups water

DIRECTIONS

1. Add all Ingredients to the slow cooker.
2. Cover the slow cooker and cook on low for 6 hours.
3. When the time has elapsed, strain and discard onions and celery. Preserve pork and cucumbers.
4. Let rest to cool then cover and refrigerate overnight.
5. Remove and discard hardened fat then warm and serve. Enjoy

NUTRITION: Calories 119, Total Fat 3g, Saturated Fat 1g, Total Carbs 0g, Net Carbs 0g, Protein 22g, Sugar: 0g, Fiber: 0g, Sodium: 50mg

Coconut Pumpkin Soup

Servings: 6

Preparation time: 10 minutes Cooking Time:
4-6 hours **INGREDIENTS**

- 1 onion, diced
- 2 cups vegetable stock
- 1 teaspoon ginger
- 1 teaspoon garlic, crushed
- ½ stick butter
- 1 pound pumpkin chunks
- 1 and 2/3 cups coconut cream
- Salt and pepper, to taste

DIRECTIONS

1. Add all the Ingredients into your slow cooker.
2. Mix them well.
3. Cook for 4-6 hours on high.
4. Puree the soup by using an immersion blender.
5. Serve and enjoy!

NUTRITION: Calories: 237; Total Fat: 21.7g; Protein: 2.4g; Carbs: 11.4g

Zucchini Soup

Servings: 4

Preparation time: 5 minutes Cooking Time:
6-8 hours **INGREDIENTS**

- A healthy soup with Zucchini as the main star.

- 4 cups vegetable broth

- 3 zucchinis, cut in chunks

- 2 tablespoons sour cream, low fat

- 2 cloves garlic, minced

- Salt, pepper, thyme, and pepper, to taste

DIRECTIONS

1. Add all the Ingredients except sour cream to a crockpot.
2. Close the lid.
3. Cook for 6-8 hours on low.
4. Add sour cream.
5. Make a smooth puree by using a blender.
6. Serve hot with parmesan cheese if you want.
7. Enjoy!

NUTRITION: Calories: 60; Total Fat: 1g; Protein: 3.5g; Carbs: 10g

Celery, Cucumber, and Zucchini Soup

Servings: 2

Preparation time: 10 minutes + 60 minutes chill time

Cooking Time: Nil

INGREDIENTS

- 3 celery stalks, chopped
- 7 ounces cucumber, cubed
- 1 tablespoon olive oil
- 2/5 cup fresh cream, 30%
- 1 red bell pepper, chopped
- 1 tablespoon dill, chopped
- 10 and ½ ounces zucchini, cubed
- Salt and pepper, to taste

DIRECTIONS

1. Put the vegetables in a juicer and juice properly.
2. Then mix in the olive oil and fresh cream.
3. Season with sauce and pepper.
4. Garnish with dill.

5. Serve it chilled and enjoy!

NUTRITION: Calories: 325; Total Fat: 32g; Protein: 4g; Carbs: 10g

Savory Cheese Soup

Servings: 6-8

Preparation time: 15 minutes

Cooking Time: 7 and ½ to 8 and ½ hours

INGREDIENTS

- 2 cups cheddar cheese, shredded
- 8 ounces cream cheese, softened
- 1/3 cup cold water
- 3 and ¾ cups vegetable broth
- 1 onion, chopped
- 1 carrot, chopped
- 1 celery, chopped
- 1/3 cup all-purpose flour
- 2 tablespoons butter
- 1 teaspoon salt
- ¼ cup red pepper, chopped
- ½ teaspoon ground pepper

DIRECTIONS

1. Add all the Ingredients except flour, cheese, and water into a crockpot.

2. Mix them well.

3. Cook the mixture for 7 to 8 hours.

4. Mix flour with water and create a smooth paste.

5. Add this to soup and cook for 30 minutes on high heat.

6. Add the cheeses and blend them well.

7. Cook for a few minutes on low.

8. Serve with croutons and enjoy!

NUTRITION: Calories: 256; Total   Fat: 20g; Protein: 9g; Carbs: 8g

Leek and Salmon Soup

Servings: 4

Preparation time: 5 minutes

Cooking Time: 3 hours and 15 minutes

INGREDIENTS

- 2 tablespoons avocado oil
- 4 leeks, washed, trimmed and sliced
- 3 garlic cloves, minced
- 2 teaspoons dried thyme leaves
- 1 pound salmon, cut into bite-sized portions
- 1 and ¾ cups of coconut milk
- Salt and pepper to taste

DIRECTIONS

1. Add avocado oil to the slow cooker pot and Set it to HIGH
2. Heat it up and add chopped up leeks, garlic and cook until tender
3. Pour stick and thyme
4. Allow the mix to simmer for 15 minutes

5. Season with some pepper and salt

6. Add coconut and salmon to the pot

7. Bring the mix to a simmer over LOW setting and keep cooking until the fish is tender for 3 hours

8. Serve!

NUTRITION: Calories: 319; Total Fat: 24g; Protein: 20g; Carbs: 4g

Chicken and Carrot Stew

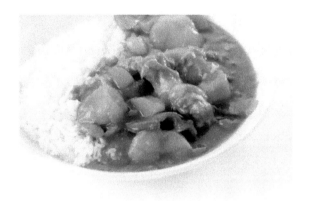

Servings: 4

Preparation time: 15 minutes Cooking

Time: 6 hours **INGREDIENTS**

- 4 chicken breast, boneless and cubed
- 2 cups chicken broth
- 1 cup tomatoes, chopped
- 3 cups carrots, peeled and cubed
- 1 teaspoon thyme, dried
- 1 cup onion, chopped
- 2 clove garlic, minced
  - Salt and pepper

DIRECTIONS

1. Add all the Ingredients to slow cooker.
2. Stir and close the lid.
3. Cook for 6 hours.
4. Serve hot and enjoy!

NUTRITION: Calories: 182; Total Fat: 3g; Protein: 39g; Carbs: 10g

Low Carb Lamb Stew

Servings: 3

Preparation time: 15 minutes Cooking Time:
6 hours **INGREDIENTS**

- 8 ounces nips, peeled and chopped
- 1 teaspoon garlic paste
- 1 teaspoon onion powder
- 14 ounces beef broth
- 1 pound lamb stewing meat, boneless
- 8 ounces mushrooms, sliced or quartered
- ¼ cup fresh flat-leaf parsley, chopped
- Salt and black pepper, to taste

DIRECTIONS

1. Add mushrooms, beef broth, lamb, turnips, onion powder, garlic paste, salt and pepper in your slow cooker.
2. Cook for about 6 hours on low.
3. Then dish out.
4. Garnish with fresh flat-leaf parsley.
5. Serve and enjoy!

NUTRITION: Calories: 360; Total Fat: 20.7g; Protein: 33g; Carbs: 8.4g

Vegetarian Garlic, Tomato & Onion Soup

Servings: 6

Preparation time: 15 minutes Cooking

Time: 30 minutes **INGREDIENTS**

- 6 cups chicken broth
- 1 teaspoon Italian seasoning
- 1 bay leaf
- ½ cup full-fat coconut milk, unsweetened
- 1 and ½ cups tomatoes, diced and canned
- 1 yellow onion, chopped
- 3 garlic cloves, peeled
- Pinch of salt and pepper, to taste

DIRECTIONS

1. Fresh basil, for serving
2. Take a stockpot and add all the Ingredients except basil and coconut milk into it.
3. Place stockpot over medium heat.
4. Let it bring to a boil.
5. Reduce heat to simmer for 30 minutes.
6. Remove the bay leaf.
7. Blend the soup until smooth by using an immersion blender

8. Add the coconut milk and stir.

9. Serve with fresh basil and enjoy!

NUTRITION: Calories: 104; Total Fat: 7g; Protein: 6g; Carbs: 7g

Celery Cucumber & Zucchini Soup

Servings: 2

Preparation time: 10 minutes + 60 minutes chill time

Cooking Time: Nil

INGREDIENTS

- 2 tablespoons olive oil
- 1 tablespoon fresh dill
- 2/5 cup fresh cream
- 7 ounces cucumber, cubed
- 10 and ½ zucchini, cubed
- 1 red pepper, chopped
- 3 celery stalks, chopped
- Salt and pepper, to taste

DIRECTIONS

1. Add all the veggies in a juice and make a smooth juice.
2. Mix in the fresh cream and olive oil.
3. Season with pepper and salt.
4. Garnish with dill.

5. Serve chilled and enjoy!

NUTRITION: Calories: 95; Total Fat: 7.6g; Protein: 2.4g; Carbs: 6.4g

Cream of Spinach Mozzarella Soup

Servings: 4

Preparation time: 10 minutes Cooking Time:
60-70 minutes

INGREDIENTS

- 2 cups chicken broth
- 1 cup mozzarella cheese, shredded
- 1 cup heavy cream
- 1 teaspoon thyme, dried
- 1 cup spinach, finely chopped
- 1 teaspoon onion powder
- 3 garlic cloves, peeled
- Salt & Black pepper, to taste

DIRECTIONS

1. Take a stockpot and add all the Ingredients except mozzarella cheese and heavy cream into it.
2. Let it bring to a boil.
3. Simmer for 60 minutes.
4. Warm the heavy cream and then add to the soup along with the mozzarella cheese.
5. Stir until the cheese has softened.

6. Serve and enjoy!

NUTRITION: Calories: 151; Total Fat: 13g; Protein: 6g; Carbs: 3g

Creamy Balsamic Tofu Stew

Servings: 4

Preparation time: 10 minutes Cooking Time:
20 minutes

INGREDIENTS

- 1 and ½ cups firm tofu, cubed
- 1 cup heavy cream
- 1 yellow onion, chopped
- 2 cups vegetable broth
- 1 green bell pepper, seeded and chopped
- ¼ cup balsamic vinegar
- 1 teaspoon garlic powder
- 1 tablespoon coconut oil, for cooking
- Salt & Black pepper, to taste

DIRECTIONS

1. Take a skillet and add the coconut oil over medium heat.

2. Then sauté the bell pepper, tofu, and onion for 10 minutes.

3. Add the balsamic, garlic powder and vegetable broth then bring to a simmer.

4. Cook for 10 minutes more or until the stew begins to thicken.

5. Season with salt and black pepper.

6. Serve and enjoy!

NUTRITION: Calories: 141; Total Fat: 8g; Protein: 11g; Carbs: 8g

Chipotle Pumpkin Soup

Servings: 6

Preparation time: 10 minutes Cooking
Time: 10-15 minutes

INGREDIENTS

- ½ cup onions
- 2 tablespoons olive oil
- 1 garlic clove, chopped
- 1 tablespoon chipotles, in adobo sauce
- 1 teaspoon ground coriander
- 1 teaspoon ground cumin
- 1/8 teaspoon ground allspice
- 2 teaspoons granulated sugar substitute
- 2 cups pumpkin puree
- 32 ounces veggie broth
- ½ cup heavy cream
- 2 teaspoons red wine vinegar
- Salt and pepper to taste

DIRECTIONS

1. Take a saucepan and place it over medium heat, add onion and garlic and Saute.

2. Mix in spices, chipotle, sugar substitute, cook for 2 minutes.

3. Mix in broth, pumpkin puree.

4. Blend until smooth using an immersion blender.

5. Mix in cream, vinegar and simmer for 5 minutes.

6. Season with salt and pepper.

7. Serve and enjoy!

NUTRITION: Calories: 138; Total Fat: 12g; Protein: 6g; Carbs: 2g

No Bean Chili

Servings: 6

Preparation time: 10 minutes Cooking Time: 40 minutes **INGREDIENTS**

- 4 cups vegetable broth
- 4 ounces tomato paste
- 1 yellow onion, chopped
- 2 cloves garlic, chopped
- ¼ cup balsamic vinegar
- 1 green bell pepper, seeded and chopped
- 2 teaspoons chili powder
- Salt & Black pepper, to taste

DIRECTIONS

1. Take a stockpot and add all the Ingredients except salt and black pepper into it.
2. Let it bring to a boil.
3. Reduce heat to simmer.
4. Cook for 40 minutes.
5. Season with salt and black pepper.
6. Serve and enjoy!

NUTRITION: Calories: 61; Total Fat: 1g; Protein: 5g; Carbs: 8g

Shrimp and Cream Soup

Servings: 4

Preparation time: 5 minutes Cooking Time: 10 minutes

INGREDIENTS

- 2 ounces shallots
- 3 ounces salmon
- 2 cups full-fat cream
- 2 ounces celery
- 3 ounces ghee
- 2 ounces clams, with juice
- 3 ounces cod
- 3 ounces shrimp
- 2 cups broth
- Salt and pepper, to taste

DIRECTIONS

1. Slice onion and celery, fry until soft.
2. Bring the broth to a boil and add seafood.
3. Reduce the heat to low and add remaining Ingredients, simmer for 10 minutes.
4. Blend the soup by using an immersion blender.

5. Serve and enjoy!

NUTRITION: Calories: 15; Total Fat: 1.7g; Protein: 2.3g; Carbs: 0g

Creamy Garlic Chicken Soup

Servings: 4

Preparation time: 10 minutes

Cooking Time: 5-10 minutes

INGREDIENTS

- 2 tablespoons butter
- 4 ounces cream cheese, cubed
- 14.5-ounce chicken broth
- 2 cups chicken, shredded
- ¼ cup heavy cream
- 2 tablespoons Stacey Hawkins Garlic Gusto Seasoning
- Salt, to taste

DIRECTIONS

1. Take a saucepan and place it over medium heat.
2. Add butter into the saucepan and melt the butter.
3. Put shredded chicken to pan and coat with melted butter.
4. Add cream cheese and Stacey Hawkins garlic gusto seasoning when chicken is warm.
5. Mix to blend the Ingredients.
6. Add chicken broth, heavy cream and evenly distributed cream cheese.

7. Bring them to boil then reduce the heat to low.

8. Simmer for 3-4 minutes.

9. Add salt to taste and serve.

10. Enjoy!

NUTRITION: Calories: 307; Total Fat: 25g; Protein: 16g; Carbs: 2g

Leftover Turkey Stew

Servings: 12

Preparation time: 10 minutes

Cooking Time: 25 minutes

INGREDIENTS

- 15 ounces can vegetables, mixed
- 2 cups turkey, cooked and cubed
- 14 ounces can chicken broth
- 3 tablespoon butter

DIRECTIONS

1. Take a saucepan and put all the Ingredients into it.
2. Bring it to boil.
3. Reduce the heat to low.
4. Simmer for about 25 minutes.
5. Dish out and serve hot.
6. Enjoy!

NUTRITION: Calories: 143; Total Fat: 6.8g; Protein: 16.2g; Carbs: 3.4g

Cheesy Beef Sausage Soup

Servings: 16

Preparation time: 30 minutes

Cooking Time: 6 hours

INGREDIENTS

- 12 ounces beer
- 14 ounces of beef smoked sausage, chopped
- 1 cup heavy cream
- 8 ounces cream cheese
- 1 teaspoon of sea salt
- ½ teaspoon black pepper
- 1 teaspoon red pepper flakes
- 32 ounces beef stock
- 2 cups sharp cheddar cheese, shredded
- 1 onion, diced
- 4 garlic cloves, minced
- 1 cup celery, chopped
- 1 cup carrots, chopped

DIRECTIONS

1. Turn on your slow cooker and add all the Ingredients except cheese and cream into it.
2. Mix them well.

3. Cover the lid.

4. Cook for 4 hours on low.

5. Now whisk in the cheese and cream.

6. Cook covered for 2 hours more.

7. Serve and enjoy!

NUTRITION: Calories: 244; Total Fat: 17g; Protein: 5g; Carbs: 4g

Creamy Subtle Broccoli Soup

Servings: 3

Preparation time: 5 minutes

Cooking Time: 35 minutes

INGREDIENTS

- 3 cups broccoli florets, chopped
- 1 can full-fat coconut milk
- ½ teaspoon onion powder
- 3 cups celery, chopped
- 2 cups vegetable stock
- ½ teaspoon garlic powder
- Red pepper flakes as needed
- Salt and pepper, to taste

DIRECTIONS

1. Take a pot and place it over medium heat.
2. Add the Ingredients to the pot.
3. Cook for about 30 minutes until the broccoli and celery are soft.
4. Transfer the soup to a blender and process them until smooth.
5. Serve hot and enjoy!

NUTRITION: Calories: 200; Total Fat: 17g; Protein: 4g; Carbs: 5g

Melon Soup

Servings: 4

Preparation time: 6 minutes

INGREDIENTS

- 4 cups casaba melon, seeded and cubed
- 1 tablespoon fresh ginger, grated
- ¾ cup of coconut milk
- Juice of 2 lime
- Salt as needed

DIRECTIONS

1. Add the lime juice, coconut milk, casaba melon, ginger and salt into your blender.
2. Blend it for 1-2 minutes until you get a smooth mixture.
3. Serve and enjoy!

NUTRITION: Calories: 134; Total Fat: 9g; Protein: 2g; Carbs: 13g

Garlic Tomato Soup

Servings: 4

Preparation time: 15 minutes Cooking
Time: 15 minutes **INGREDIENTS**

- 8 Roma tomatoes, chopped
- 1 cup tomatoes, sundried
- 2 tablespoons coconut oil
- ¾ teaspoon Himalayan pink salt
- 5 cloves garlic, chopped
- 14 ounces coconut milk, full-fat
- 1 cup vegetable broth
- Ground black pepper, to taste

DIRECTIONS

1. Basil, for garnish
2. Take a pot, heat oil into it.
3. Sauté the garlic in it for ½ minute.
4. Mix in the Roma tomatoes and cook for 8-10 minutes.
5. Stir occasionally.
6. Add in the rest of the Ingredients except the basil and stir well.
7. Cover the lid and cook for 5 minutes.
8. Let it cool.

9. Blend the soup until smooth by using an immersion blender.

10. Garnish with basil.

11. Serve and enjoy!

NUTRITION: Calories: 233.6; Total Fat: 23.4g; Protein: 4g; Carbs: 16.1g

Clam Chowder

Servings: 8

Preparation time: 10 minutes Cooking Time:
4-6 hours **INGREDIENTS**

- 2 cans whole baby clams, with juice
- 2 cups whipping cream, heavy
- 13 slices bacon, thickly cut
- 2 cups chicken broth
- 1 cup onion, chopped
- 1 cup celery, chopped
- 1 teaspoon thyme, grounded
- 1 teaspoon salt
- 1 teaspoon pepper

DIRECTIONS

1. Take a skillet and place the bacon into it.
2. Cook the bacon till it becomes crispy.
3. Remove and let it cool then crumble it.
4. Sauté the onion and celery in the bacon grease.
5. Turn on your slow cooker and transfer them.
6. Combine the rest of the Ingredients in a slow cooker.
7. Cover the lid.

8. Cook for 4-6 hours on low.

9. Serve and enjoy!

NUTRITION: Calories: 427; Total Fat: 33g; Protein: 27g; Carbs: 5g

Pumpkin, Coconut & Sage Soup

Servings: 6

Preparation time: 15 minutes Cooking Time: 30 minutes **INGREDIENTS**

- 1 cup pumpkin, canned
- 6 cups chicken broth
- 1 cup full-fat coconut milk
- 1 teaspoon sage, freshly chopped
- 3 garlic cloves, peeled
- Pinch of salt and pepper, to taste

DIRECTIONS

1. Take a stockpot and add all the Ingredients except coconut milk into it.
2. Place stockpot over medium heat.
3. Let it bring to a boil.
4. Reduce heat to simmer for 30 minutes.
5. Add the coconut milk and stir.
6. Serve bacon and enjoy!

NUTRITION: Calories: 146;   Total Fat: 11g; Protein: 6g; Carbs: 7g

Rosemary and Thyme Cucumber Soup

Servings: 6

Preparation time: 10 minutes + 60 minutes chill time

Cooking Time: nil

INGREDIENTS

- 4 cups vegetable broth
- 1 teaspoon thyme, freshly chopped
- 1 teaspoon rosemary, freshly chopped
- 2 cucumbers, sliced
- 1 cup heavy cream
- 1 pinch of salt

DIRECTIONS

1. Take a large mixing bowl and add all the Ingredients into it.
2. Whisk them well.
3. Blend until smooth by using an immersion blender.
4. Let it chill for 1 hour.
5. Serve and enjoy!

NUTRITION: Calories: 111; Total Fat: 9g; Protein: 5g; Carbs: 4g

Cream of Zucchini Soup

Servings: 4

Preparation time: 5 minutes Cooking Time: 20 minutes **INGREDIENTS**

- ½ small onion, quartered
- 2 cloves garlic
- Parmesan cheese, freshly grated
- 2 tablespoons sour cream, fat-free
- 32-ounce Swanson chicken broth, low sodium
- Kosher salt and black pepper, to taste

DIRECTIONS

1. Take a pot and place it over medium heat.
2. Add onion, chicken broth, zucchini, and garlic into the pot.
3. Bring them to boil.
4. Reduce the heat and cover the lid.
5. Simmer for 20 minutes or until tender.
6. Remove from the heat and puree by using an immersion blender.
7. Add sour cream and puree again until you get a smooth mixture.
8. Add salt and pepper to taste and serve.

9. Enjoy!

NUTRITION: Calories: 60; Total Fat: 1g; Protein: 3.5g; Carbs: 10g

Cream of Mushroom Soup

Servings: 4

Preparation time: 5 minutes Cooking
Time: 6 hours **INGREDIENTS**

- 20 ounces mushrooms, sliced
- 1 cup heavy cream
- 2 cups chicken broth
- 1 cup almond milk, unsweetened
- Salt, garlic, onion powder, and pepper, to taste

DIRECTIONS

1. Add all Ingredients to a crockpot.
2. Close the lid.
3. Cook for 6 hours on low.
4. Make a smooth puree by using a blender.
5. Serve hot and enjoy!

NUTRITION: Calories: 229; Total Fat: 23g; Protein: 5g; Carbs: 7

Spicy Pork Stew and Spinach

Servings: 6

Preparation time: 10 minutes Cooking Time:

25 minutes **INGREDIENTS**

- 4 garlic cloves

- 1 large onion

- 1 teaspoon thyme, dried

- 1 pound pork butt meat, cut into 2 inch chunks

- 4 cups baby spinach, chopped

- 2 teaspoons Cajun seasoning blend

- ½ cup heavy whip cream

DIRECTIONS

1. Blend garlic, onion, and transfer to a pressure cooker.

2. Add Cajun seasoning blend, pork and lock lid.

3. Cook for 20 minutes at HIGH pressure.

4. Release pressure naturally over 10 minutes, stir in baby spinach and cream.

5. Let them Saute for 5 minutes. Serve!

NUTRITION: Calories: 376;   Total Fat: 24g; Protein: 20g; Carbs: 5g

Thai Pumpkin Seafood Stew

Servings: 4

Preparation time: 5 minutes Cooking Time:

35 minutes **INGREDIENTS**

- 1 and ½ tablespoons fresh galangal, roughly chopped
- 1 teaspoon lime zest
- 1 small Kabocha squash
- 32 medium-sized mussels, fresh
- 1 pound shrimp
- 16 leave Thai leaves
- 1 can (14 ounces coconut milk
- 1 tablespoon lemongrass, minced
- 4 garlic cloves, roughly chopped
- 32 medium-sized clams, fresh
- 1 and ½ pounds fresh salmon
- 2 tablespoons coconut oil
- Salt and pepper to taste

DIRECTIONS

1. Add coconut milk, lemongrass, galangal, garlic, lime leaves in a small-sized saucepan, bring to a boil.
2. Let it simmer for 25 minutes.
3. Strain mixture through fine sieve into the large soup pot

and bring to a simmer.

4. Add oil to a pan and heat up, add Kabocha squash.

5. Season with salt and pepper, Saute for 5 minutes.

6. Add mix to coconut mix.

7. Heat oil in a pan and add fish shrimp, season with salt and pepper, cook for 4 minutes.

8. Add mixture to coconut milk mix alongside clams and mussels.

9. Simmer for 8 minutes, garnish with basil and enjoy!

NUTRITION: Calories: 389; Total Fat: 16g; Protein: 48g; Carbs: 10g

Garlicky Chicken Soup

Servings: 6

Preparation time: 10 minutes Cooking
Time: 15 minutes **INGREDIENTS**

- 2 chicken breast, boneless and skinless
- 4 cups chicken broth
- 1 teaspoon thyme
- 1 tablespoon butter, for cooking
- 1 cup heavy cream
- 3 garlic cloves, peeled
- 1 teaspoon salt
- ¼ teaspoon black pepper

DIRECTIONS

1. Take a stockpot and preheat it over medium heat with the butter.
2. Add the chicken and brown until completely cooked through.
3. Remove the heat.
4. Shred the chicken and add it back to the stockpot nearby whatever is left of the fixings except for the cream cheddar.
5. Let it bring to a simmer.

6. Add the cream cheese and whisk properly.

7. Simmer for 10 minutes.

8. Serve bacon and enjoy!

NUTRITION: Calories: 120; Total Fat: 6g; Protein: 16g; Carbs: 2g

Bacon Cabbage Chuck Beef Stew

Servings: 6

Preparation time: 10 minutes Cooking Time: 7
hours **INGREDIENTS**

- A meaty and healthy stew for any lunch or dinner, the combination of bacon and cabbage offers a very subliminal yet satisfying flavor.
- 1 cup beef bone broth, homemade
- ½ pound bacon
- 2 small red onion, peeled and sliced
- 2 pounds grass-fed chuck roast, cut in 2" pieces
- 1 small Napa cabbage
- 1 garlic clove, minced
- 1 spring thyme, fresh
- Salt and black pepper, to taste

DIRECTIONS

1. Add bacon slices, garlic and onion slices at the bottom of the slow cooker.
2. Layer with the chuck roast, following by the cabbage slices, thyme, and broth.

3. Season with salt and black pepper.

4. Cook on low for 7 hours.

5. Once cooked, dish out.

6. Serve hot and enjoy!

NUTRITION: Calories: 170; Total Fat: 9g; Protein: 19.5g; Carbs: 3.4g

The Kale and Spinach Soup

Servings: 4

Preparation time: 5 minutes Cooking
Time: 5 minutes **INGREDIENTS**

- 8 ounces kale, chopped
- 2 avocados, diced
- 4 and 1/3 cups of coconut milk
- 3 ounces of coconut oil
- Salt and pepper to taste

DIRECTIONS

1. Take a skillet and place it over medium heat.
2. Add kale and sauté for 2-3 minutes.
3. Then add kale to your blender.
4. Put spices, coconut milk, water, and avocado to the blender as well.
5. Blend until smooth and pour mixture into a bowl.
6. Serve and enjoy!

NUTRITION: Calories: 124;   Total   Fat: 13g;   Protein: 4.2g;
Carbs: 7g

Beef Bone Broth

Preparation Time: 10 minutes

Cooking time 8 hours Servings: 8

INGREDIENTS

- 2 lbs. Rumba meats beef hid shank
- ½ lb. Rumba meats marrowbone
- ½ tbsp kosher salt
- 1 tbsp olive oil
- 2 cucumbers, unpeeled and cut into pieces
- 1 onion, unpeeled and quartered
- 1 garlic head, unpeeled
- 1 green pepper, cut into pieces
- 2 celery stalks, cut into pieces
- 1 leek, cut into pieces
- 1 tbsp beef bouillon
- 2 bay leaves
- 7 peppercorns
- 8 cups water
- 2 tbsp apple cider vinegar

DIRECTIONS

1. Season hind shank and bones with salt and pepper
2. Heat oil in a nonstick skillet then brown the shank and bones on all sides. Transfer to a slow cooker.

3. Add cucumbers, onions, pepper, celery stalks, leek, beef bouillon, bay leaves, peppercorns, and salt to the slow cooker.
4. Add water until the veggies and bones are submerged.
5. Cover the slow cooker and cook on low for 8 hours.
6. When the time has elapsed, let rest to cool. Use a fine-mesh sieve to strain the broth.
7. Discard vegetables and bones and let continue resting to cool. Remove fat from the top if any.
8. Serve and enjoy.

NUTRITION: Calories 78, Total Fat 6g, Saturated Fat 1g, Total Carbs 5g, Net Carbs 4g, Protein 1g, Sugar: 2g, Fiber: 1g, Sodium: 477mg, Potassium: 140mg

Chicken Feet Bone broth

Preparation Time: 5 minutes

Cooking time 12 hours Servings: 8

INGREDIENTS

- 12 chicken feet, pastured
- 16 cups water, filtered
- 1 tbsp salt
- 1 sprig rosemary
- ½ inch fresh ginger

DIRECTIONS

1. Add chicken feet, with the outer membrane removed, to the slow cooker.
2. Add water until the feet are submerged. Cover the slow cooker and bring it to boil.
3. Use a spoon to skim off any fat on top. Add salt, rosemary, and ginger then cook on low for 12 hours.
4. When the time has elapsed, let the broth rest to cool.
   5. Strain the broth in jars then serve and enjoy.

NUTRITION: Calories 103, Total Fat 5.9g, Saturated Fat 1.75g, Total Carbs 1.8g, Net Carbs 1.8g, Protein 10.6g, Sugar: 0g, Fiber: 0g, Sodium: 683mg, Potassium: 411mg

Gingery High Collagen Bone Broth

Preparation Time: 30 minutes

Cooking time 10 hours Servings: 8

INGREDIENTS

- 2 lbs. chicken wings, cut into pieces
- 1 lb. chicken feet
- 1 onion
- 1 cucumber
- 1 stalk celery
- 8 garlic cloves, minced
- 1 inch ginger, minced
- 1 tbsp salt
- ½ tbsp black pepper
- 4 cups water

DIRECTIONS

- Add all Ingredients to the slow cooker. The water should submerge all the Ingredients.
- Cover and cook on high for 10 hours.
- When the time has elapsed, strain the broth in a fine mesh strainer then discard the solids.
- You may store the broth in food storage containers or

serve and enjoy.

NUTRITION: Calories 262, Total Fat 18g, Saturated Fat 4g, Total Carbs 3g, Net Carbs 3g, Protein 22g, Sugar: 1g, Fiber: 0g, Sodium: 390mg, Potassium: 182mg

Nacho Cheese Sauce Cheese Sauce

Preparation Time: 5 minutes

Cooking time 11 hour; Serves 16

INGREDIENTS

- 16 oz cheddar cheese, extra sharp
- 2 tbsp chia seeds
- 2 cans full-fat milk
- 1 tbsp. Franks Red hot sauce

DIRECTIONS

1. Add all the Ingredients to the slow cooker.
2. Cover the slow cooker and cook on low for 1 to 2 hours
3. When the time has elapsed, give a good stir.
4. Serve and enjoy when warm. Add all the Ingredients to the slow cooker.
5. Cover the slow cooker and cook on low for 1 to 2 hours. When the time has elapsed, stir well.
6. Leave on keep warm setting then serve and enjoy.

NUTRITION: Calories 172, Total Fat 12.2g, Saturated Fat 88g, Total Carbs 5.5g, Net Carbs 5.5g, Protein 10.10g, Sugar: 04g, Fiber: 00g, Sodium: 2512mg, Potassium: 1611mg

Creamy Keto Cheese Sauce

Preparation Time: 5 minutes

Cooking time 1 hour;

Serves 8

INGREDIENTS

- 1 cup heavy cream
- 4 oz sharp cheddar cheese, grated
- 2 tbsp Dijon mustard

DIRECTIONS

1. Add all the Ingredients to the slow cooker.
2. Cover the slow cooker and cook on low for 1 to 2 hours.
3. When the time has elapsed, stir well.
4. Serve and enjoy.

NUTRITION: Calories 155, Total Fat 15g, Saturated Fat 9g, Total Carbs 1g, Net Carbs 1g, Protein 4g, Sugar: 0g, Fiber: 0g, Sodium: 113mg, Potassium: 36mg

Tarragon Mushroom Sauce

Preparation Time: 10 minutes

Cooking time 2 hours Servings: 4

INGREDIENTS

- 1 tbsp butter
- 1 garlic clove, crushed
- 1 onion, thinly sliced
- ½ tbsp salt
- Pinch pepper, ground
- 7 oz mushrooms, thinly sliced
- 5 tbsp Worcestershire sauce
- 1 tbsp Dijon mustard
- ½ cup heavy cream
- 2 tbsp tarragon, fresh and finely chopped

DIRECTIONS

1. Heat a skillet over high heat and sauté butter, garlic clove, onions, salt, and ground pepper until the onions are translucent.

2. Add mushrooms and cook for 3minutes. Transfer to a slow cooker.

3. Add all other Ingredients except tarragon, cover the slow

cooker and cook on low for 2 hours.

4. Stir in tarragon and serve. Enjoy.

NUTRITION: Calories 166, Total Fat 14g, Saturated Fat 8g, Total Carbs 7g, Net Carbs 4g, Protein 3g, Sugar: 2g, Fiber: 3g, Sodium: 448mg, Potassium: 371mg

Italian Meat Sauce

Preparation Time: 5 minutes

Cooking time 2 hours

Servings: 8

INGREDIENTS

- ¾ lb. beef, grass-fed and ground
- ½ lb. sweet Italian sausage
- Olive oil
- 1 garlic clove, minced
- ⅓ cup white wine
- 28 oz organic crushed tomatoes, no salt
- 1 tbsp basil, fresh
- Salt and pepper

DIRECTIONS

1. Brown beef and sausage in a nonstick skillet over medium heat.
2. Add oil and sauté garlic for 20 seconds ensuring it doesn't burn.
3. Deglaze the skillet with wine. Scrap up all the brown bits then transfer to a slow cooker.
4. Add all other Ingredients, cover the slow cooker and

cook on low for 1 ½ hours.

5. Serve and enjoy over zoodles or spaghetti squash.

NUTRITION: Calories 200, Total Fat 12g, Saturated Fat 4g, Total Carbs 7g, Net Carbs 4g, Protein 16g, Sugar: 3g, Fiber: 3g

Pepper Sauce

Preparation Time: 5 minutes

Cooking time 2 hours Servings: 4

INGREDIENTS

- 1 tbsp butter
- ½ onion, finely diced
- 1 cup beef stock
- ½ cup heavy cream
- 2 tbsp green peppercorns
- ¼ tbsp black pepper, coarsely ground
- ¼ tbsp white pepper, ground
- ½ tbsp xanthan gum
- Salt to taste

DIRECTIONS

1. Sauté butter and onions in a skillet over high heat until the onions are translucent.
2. Add stock and cook until it's reduced by half.
3. Transfer to a slow cooker and add cream and peppers.
4. Cover and cook on low for 1 hour. Sprinkle xanthan gum, salt, and pepper then stir well.
5. Adjust salt and serve over vegetables or chicken.

NUTRITION: Calories 137, Total Fat 13g, Saturated Fat 8g, Total Carbs 3g, Net Carbs 2g, Protein 2g, Sugar: 0g, Fiber: 1g, Sodium: 313mg, Potassium: 153mg

Buffalo Wing Sauce

Preparation Time: 5 minutes

Cooking time 1 hour; serves 6

INGREDIENTS

- ⅔ cup Franks Red Hot pepper sauce
- cup butter, unsalted
- 1 ½ tbsp white vinegar
- ¼ tbsp Worcestershire sauce

DIRECTIONS

1. Add all Ingredients in a slow cooker.
2. Give a good stir, cover and cook on low for 1 hour or until bubbling.
3. Serve and enjoy.

NUTRITION: Calories 151, Total Fat 15g, Saturated Fat 9g, Total Carbs 0g, Net Carbs 0g, Protein 4g, Sugar: 0g, Fiber: 0g, Sodium: 709mg, Potassium: 38mg

Bolognese Sauce

Preparation Time: 10 minutes

Cooking time: 8 hours 50 minutes

Servings: 8

INGREDIENTS

- 2 lbs. beef, ground
- 2 finely chopped onions, large
- 2 finely chopped cucumbers
- 5 minced garlic cloves
- 1 cup tomato paste, unsalted
- 2 beef stock cubes
- 1 cup water, boiling for stock cubes
- 1 tbsp sea salt
- 4 chopped and skinned tomatoes, fresh
- ½ cup melted ghee
- 1 tbsp almond flour, thinned paste using water

DIRECTIONS

1. Place ghee on a heavy skillet then caramelize onions over medium heat until soft.

2. Add garlic and fry for about 1-2 minutes then transfer into a slow cooker bowl.

3. Brown beef in the skillet over high heat. Cook in batches transferring into the slowcooker and avoiding meat from being stewed.

4. Add tomatoes, dissolved stock cubes, cucumbers, and tomato paste into your slow cooker then use a spoon, wooden, to mix

thoroughly.

5. Cook for about 30 minutes on high until a hot sauce.

6. Lower heat to low and cook for about 7-8 hours. Check for meat sauce consistency

   1 hour before turning off your slow cooker.

7. Add flour paste, almond, if the sauce is thin then stir occasionally during the last hour.

8. Serve over zucchini noodles and splash with cheese, parmesan.

9. Use a crispy salad and voila as a side for a perfect keto.

10. Enjoy!

NUTRITION: Calories: 430, Total Fat: 27.5g, Saturated 11.3g, Total Carbs: 10.8g, Net Carbs: 8.3g, Protein: 34.7g, Sugars: 5.2g, Fiber: 2.5g, Sodium: 385mg, Potassium: 673mg

CPSIA information can be obtained
at www.ICGtesting.com
Printed in the USA
BVHW042008110321
602277BV00007B/501